"To my son Brandon. Thank you for making me the person I am today."

- Much love, Mom

"To my loving wife Yu Yuan, my son Julian, and my daughters Caitlyn and Kara, with love. Furthermore, to my parents, and my sisters for forever supporting my creative endeavors."

- Alex T. Lee

Perfect

A Journey of CMV, Love and Resiliency

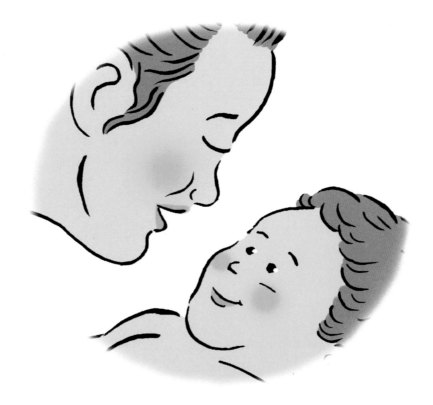

By Patty Cutshall-Bailey

Illustrated by Alexander T. Lee

You were safe inside me, all snuggled and warm. I was protecting you from everything, saving you from harm.

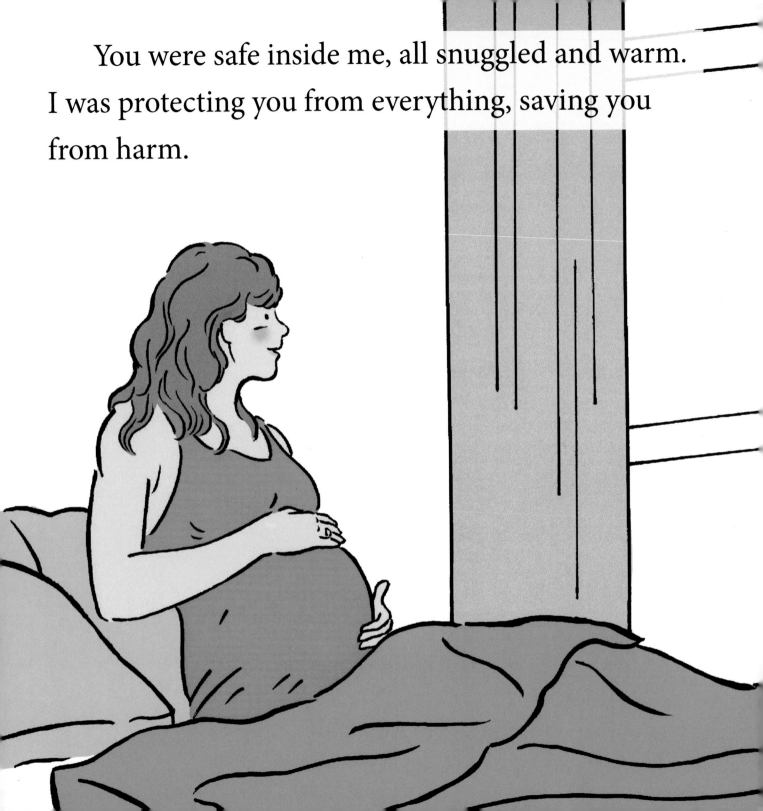

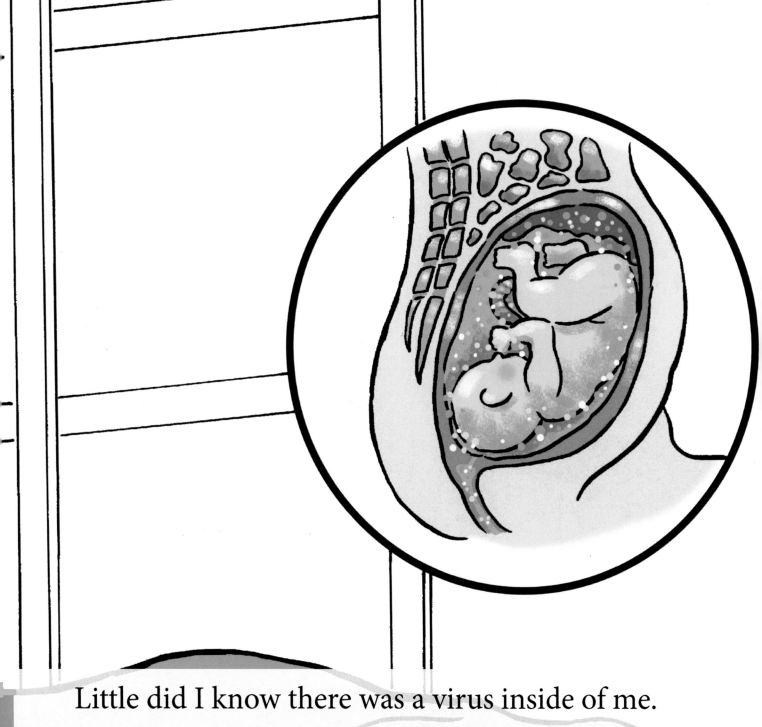

Little did I know there was a virus inside of me.

It was causing damage, but I didn't know, I couldn't see.

Intrauterine Growth Retardation the doctor determined. On the screen we could see that your growth was disrupted. Amniocentesis proved your lungs were developed, you were delivered by c-section early, and just like that my world erupted.

Your head was so small; it could fit right in my hand.

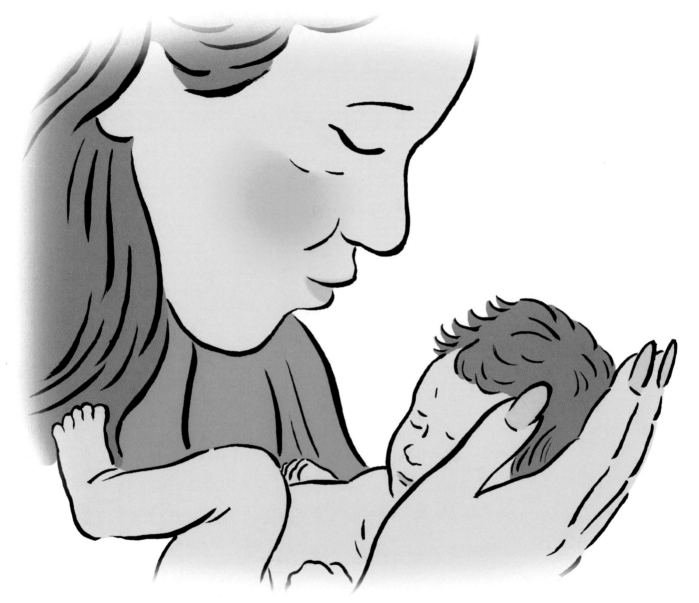

Although all seemed normal, what came next was unplanned.

After 36 hours the seizures began; you wouldn't go home. Not without probing; not without scans.

MRIs, EKGs, blood tests galore. Would they find a reason? Could they do more? For nine days you endured tests to answer these questions. To me you were perfect, why all the interventions?

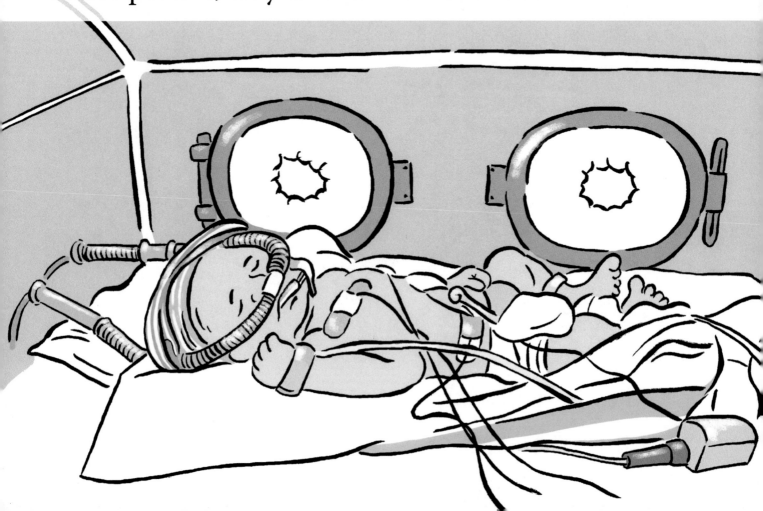

I listened to them predict; I listened to them heed. "I'm the best thing for my son," I said, "I'm all that he needs."

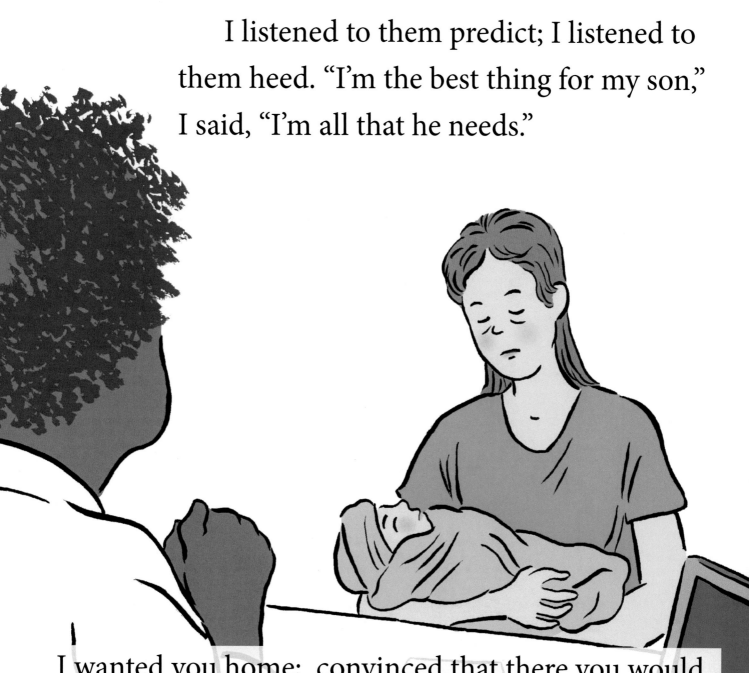

I wanted you home; convinced that there you would thrive. I was sure that I was all you needed to stay alive.

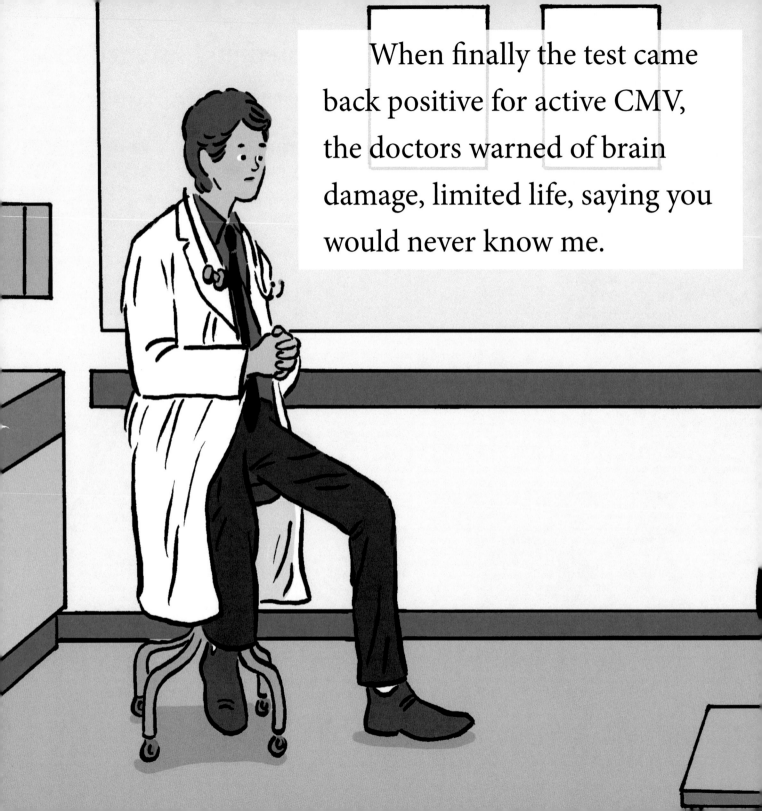

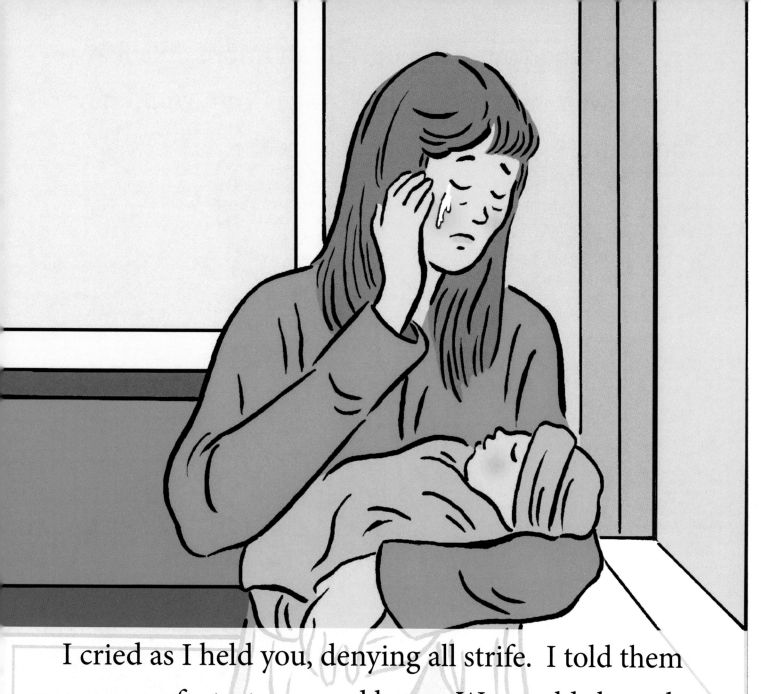

I cried as I held you, denying all strife. I told them you were perfect, strong and brave. We would show those doctors; you would never be depraved.

Holding your head up was an impossible feat. There were many other milestones you would never quite meet.

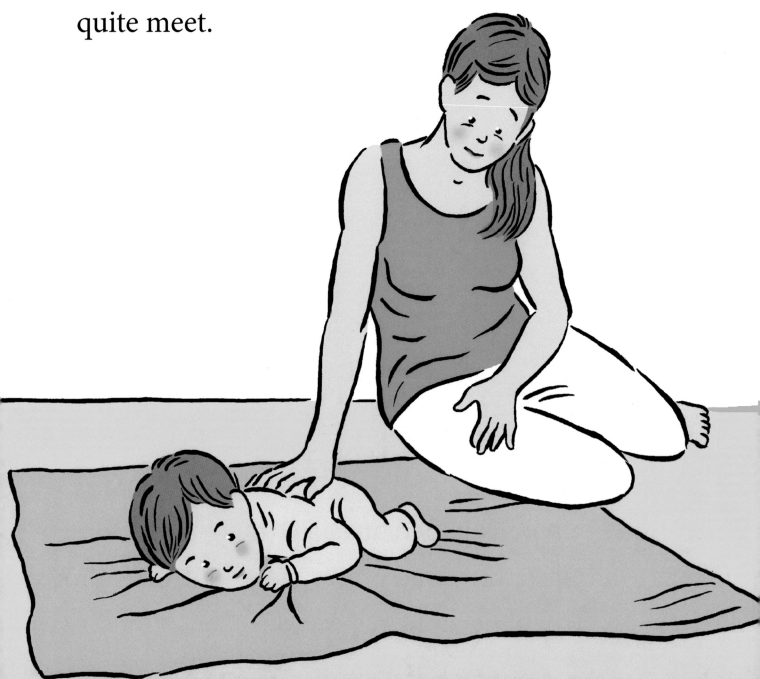

At two years old, you still were the size of a baby. Feeding was hard; it was driving me crazy. The doctors suggested a tube in your belly. Real food was not an option; you would never have peanut butter and jelly.

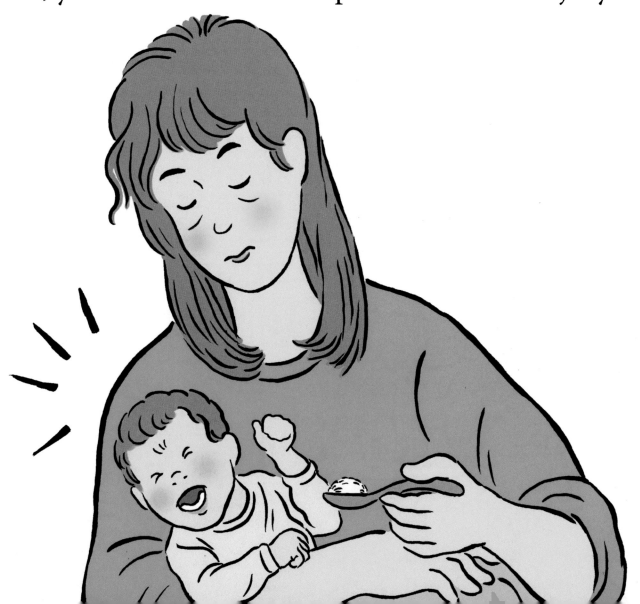

Your body would start growing, but your bones just couldn't settle. No standing, nor running; it would make things detrimental.   You had hip surgeries and heel releases that wouldn't help you step; but they provided some comfort, lessened the pain and gave you your pep.

Although you would coo and make noise with your voice, saying 'I love you' or 'mom' wasn't a choice.

You would speak with your eyes; you would speak with your grin. I knew what you needed and I would always give in.

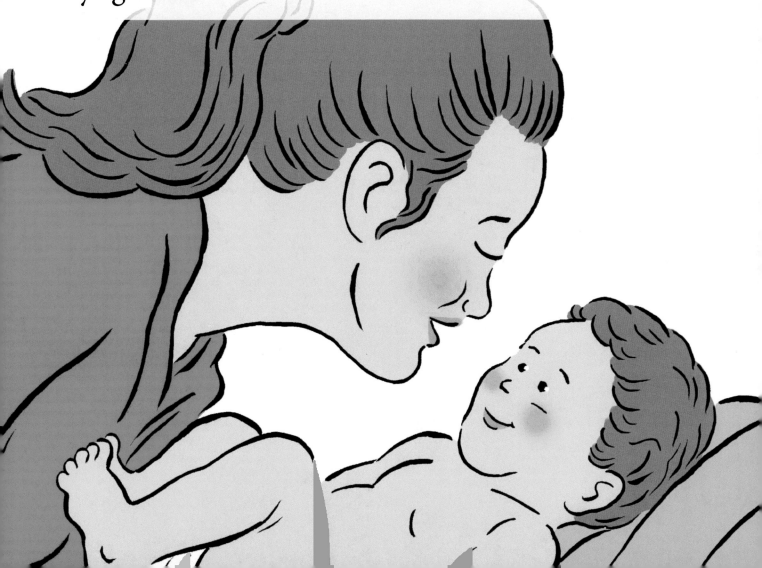

Finding caregivers was a battle; they just couldn't see. Caring for you wasn't typical, and it couldn't always be me.

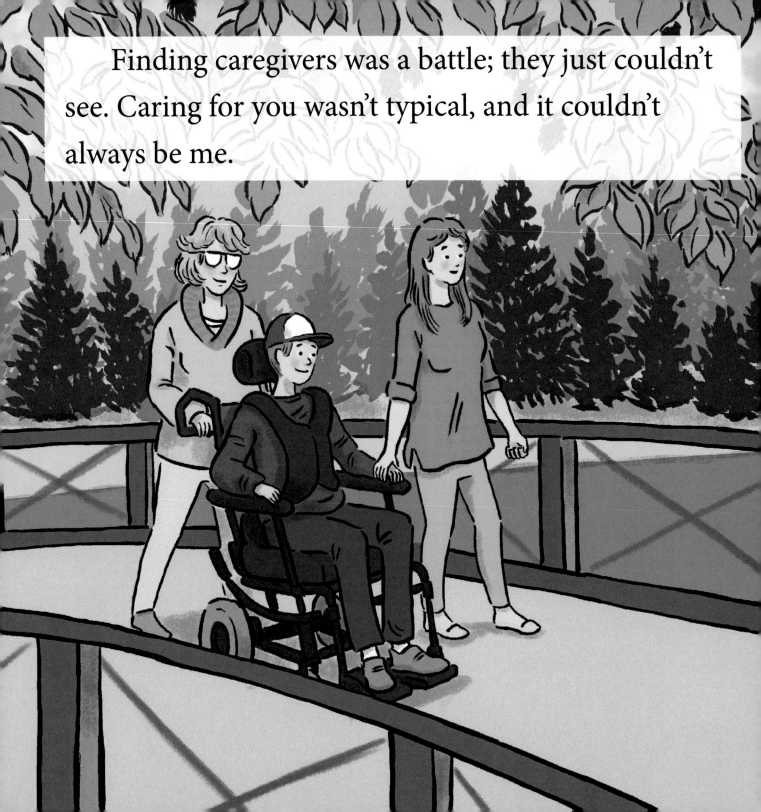

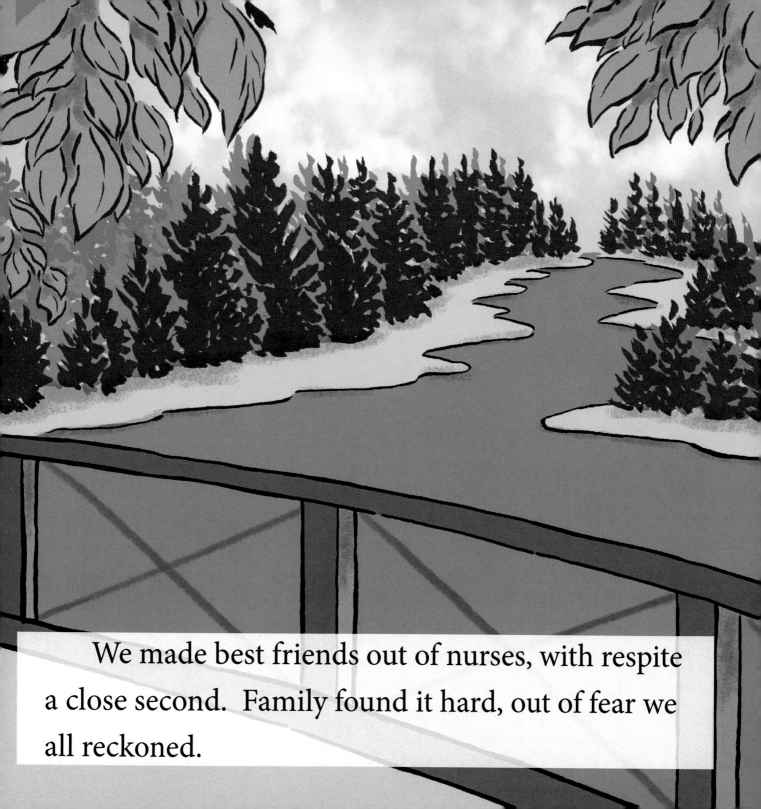

We made best friends out of nurses, with respite a close second. Family found it hard, out of fear we all reckoned.

Birthdays were different since you couldn't eat cake. Each one would come with gloom; each one made my heart ache. I wanted you to have everything; I wanted you to thrive. But I was doing all I could, I was keeping you alive.

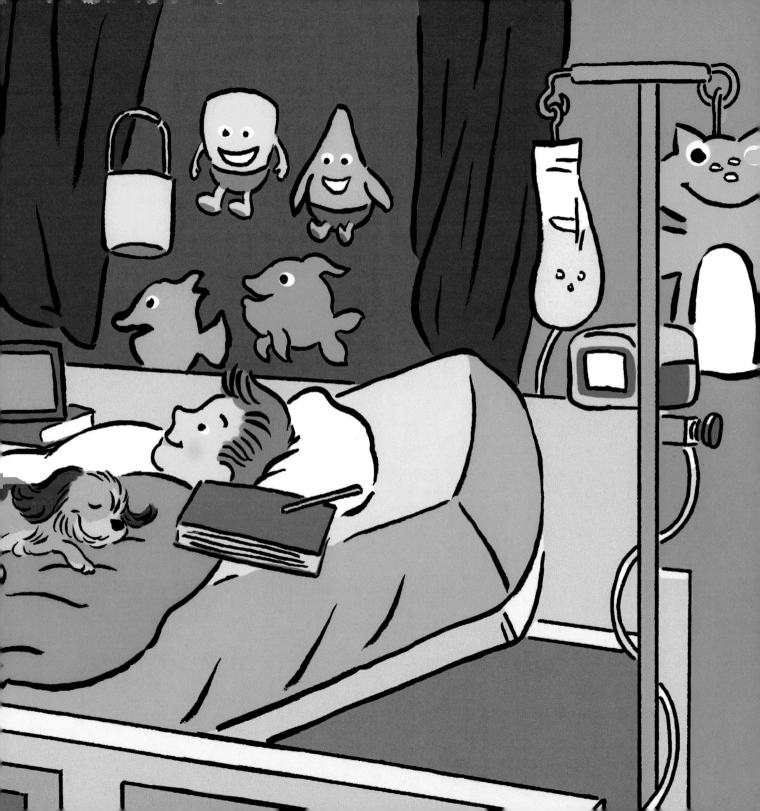

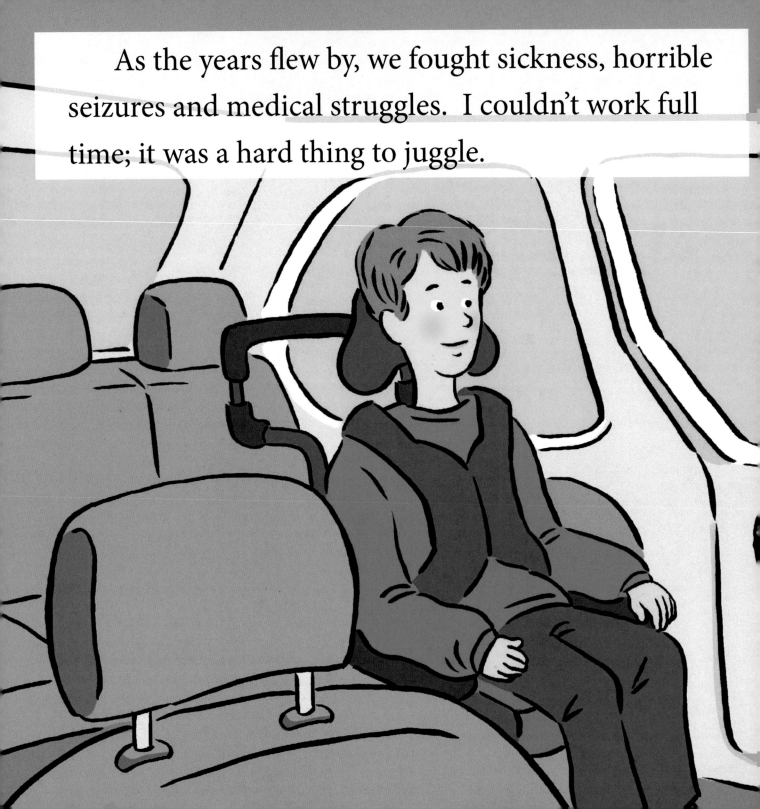

As the years flew by, we fought sickness, horrible seizures and medical struggles. I couldn't work full time; it was a hard thing to juggle.

Appointments were vital, there were experts to see. OT, PT, and Speech were important to the thousandth degree.

I loved you, you see, and you were my responsibility.

Until one day I woke up and wondered about your possibilities. You were my life, and I was yours. Was there something we were missing? Was I holding you back? Were we really living?

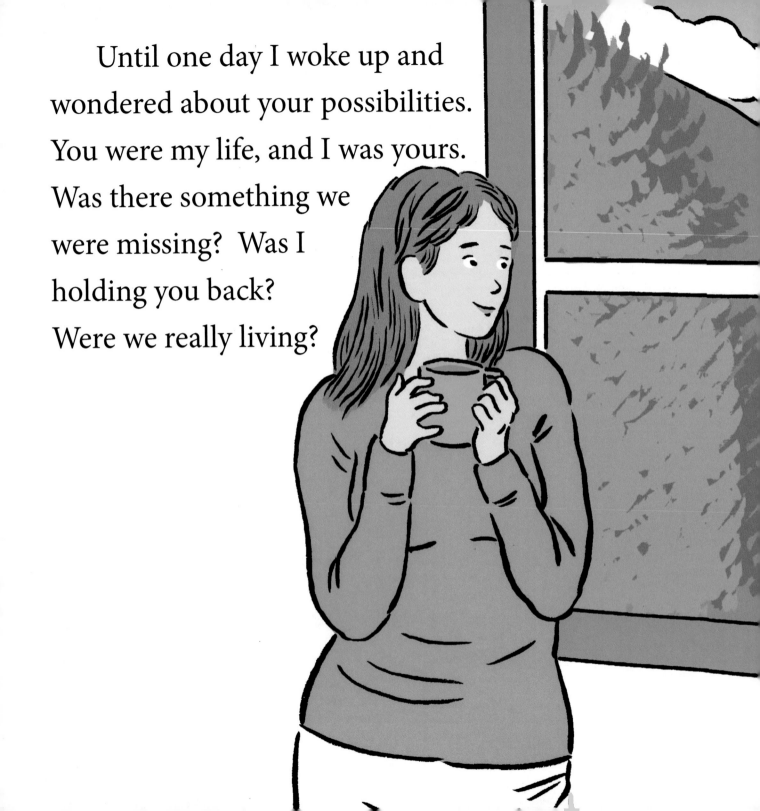

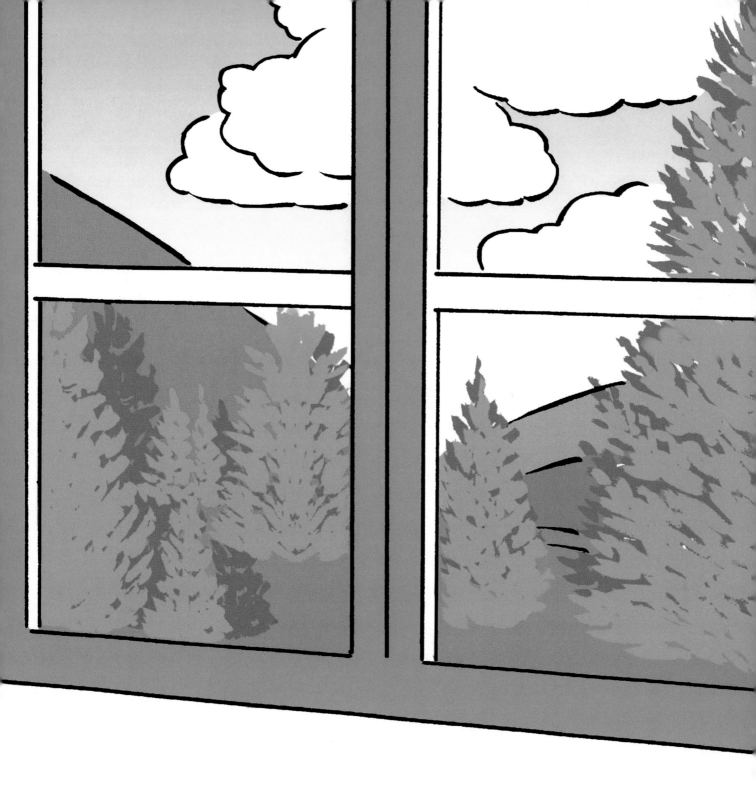

Moving you from home and from all of those who loved you was a very hard decision, a difficult choice to make.

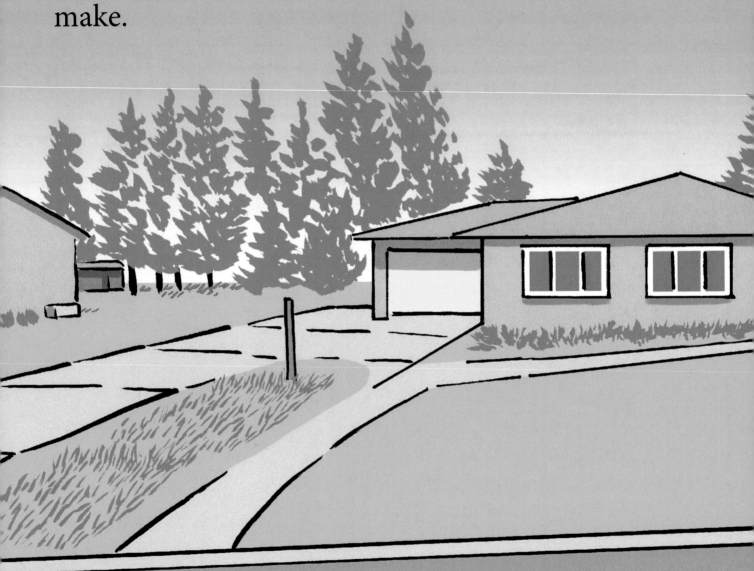

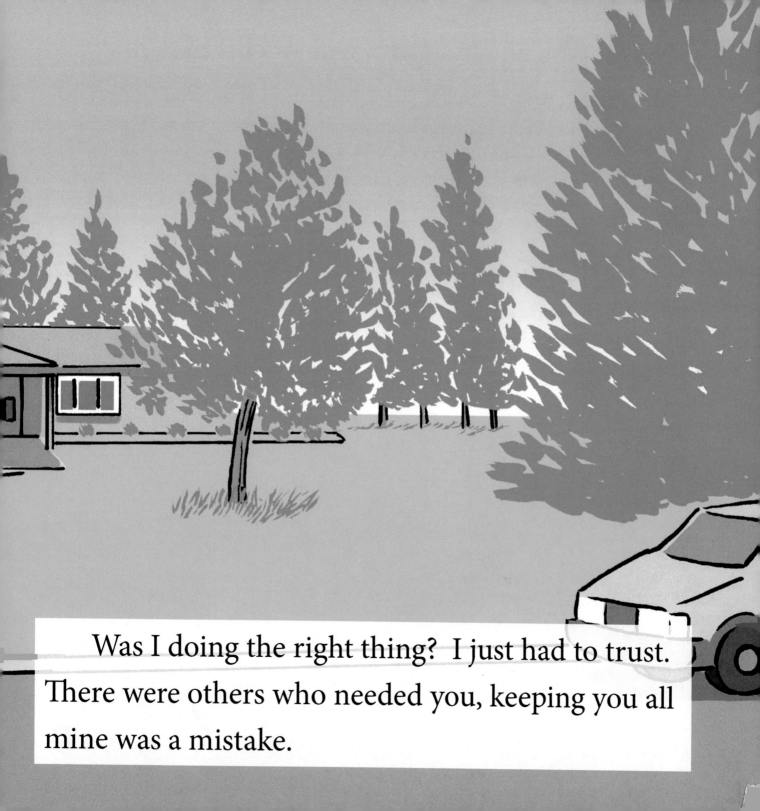

Was I doing the right thing? I just had to trust.
There were others who needed you, keeping you all
mine was a mistake.

You won't have a job, a wife or children, but you will have opportunities and a good life worth living.

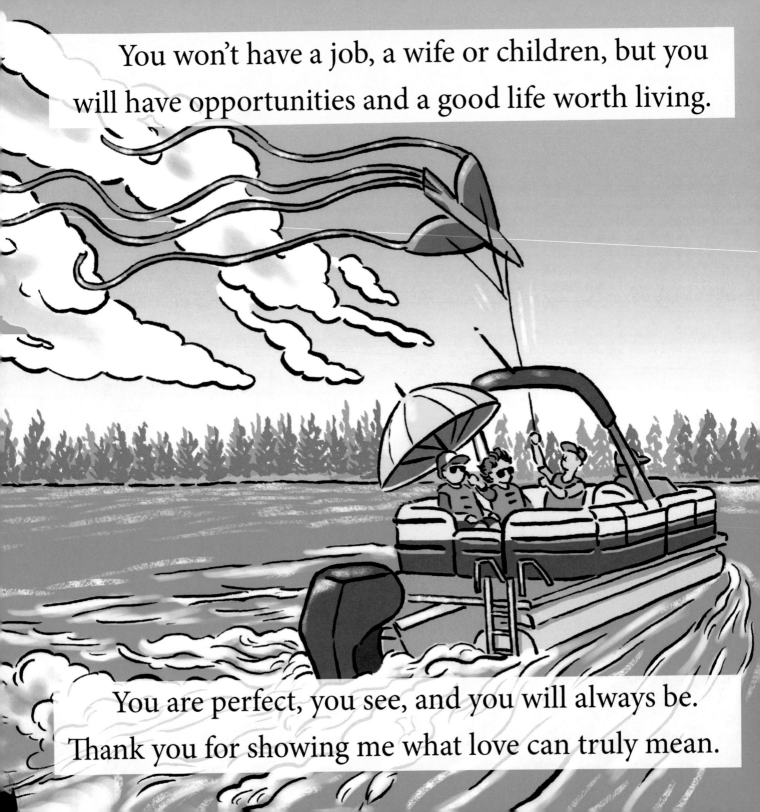

You are perfect, you see, and you will always be. Thank you for showing me what love can truly mean.

Note for the Reader:
Hello! As you are reading this story, there may be some words that are long and hard for your kiddo to understand. Feel free to give the definition or meaning of the words if asked. I have included them here for easy reference:

CMV: Cytomegalovirus infection is a common herpesvirus infection.

Intrauterine Growth Retardation: IUGR is a term that's used to describe a baby who isn't growing as quickly as he should be inside the womb.

Amniocentesis: Amniocentesis is a procedure in which amniotic fluid is removed from the uterus for testing or treatment. Amniotic fluid is the fluid that surrounds and protects a baby during pregnancy.

MRI: Magnetic resonance imaging (MRI) is a medical imaging technique that uses a magnetic field and computer-generated radio waves to create detailed images of the organs and tissues in your body. It can be used to detect brain tumors, traumatic brain injury, developmental anomalies, multiple sclerosis, stroke, dementia, infection, and the causes of headache.

EKG: An electrocardiogram (**ECG** or **EKG**) records the electrical signal from your heart to check for different heart conditions.

Made in the USA
Columbia, SC
28 January 2022

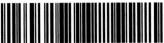
54937218R00020